T0043428

AN ANTHOLOGY OF MONSTERS

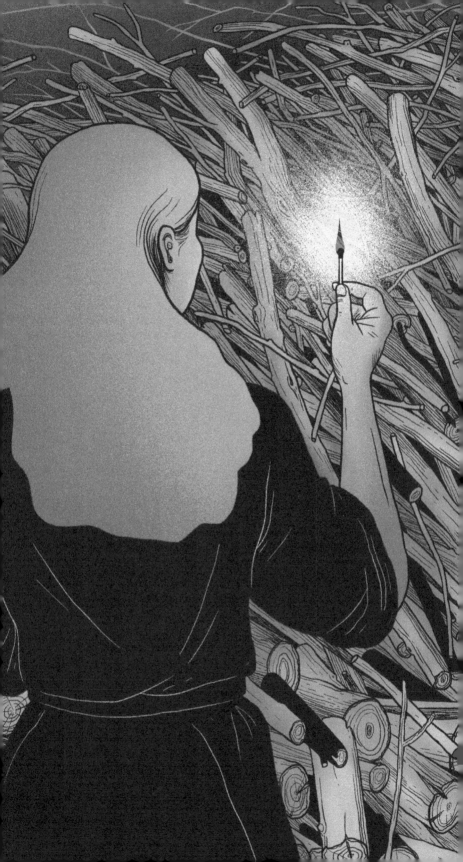

CLC KREISEL LECTURE SERIES

CHERIE DIMALINE

AN ANTHOLOGY OF MONSTERS

HOW STORY SAVES US FROM OUR ANXIETY

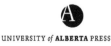

UNIVERSITY *of* ALBERTA PRESS

Canadian Literature Centre
Centre de littérature canadienne

PUBLISHED BY

University of Alberta Press
1-16 Rutherford Library South
11204 89 Avenue NW
Edmonton, Alberta, Canada T6G 2J4
amiskwaciwâskahikan | Treaty 6 |
Métis Territory
uap.ualberta.ca | uapress@ualberta.ca

and

Canadian Literature Centre /
Centre de littérature canadienne
3-5 Humanities Centre
University of Alberta
Edmonton, Alberta, Canada T6G 2E5
www.abclc.ca

Copyright © 2023 Cherie Dimaline

LIBRARY AND ARCHIVES CANADA
CATALOGUING IN PUBLICATION

Title: An anthology of monsters :
    how story saves us from our anxiety /
    Cherie Dimaline.
Names: Dimaline, Cherie, 1975– author.
Series: Henry Kreisel lecture series.
Description: Series statement: CLC
    Kreisel lecture
Identifiers: Canadiana (print)
    2022046751X | Canadiana (ebook)
    20220467900 | ISBN 9781772126822
    (softcover) | ISBN 9781772126860
    (EPUB) | ISBN 9781772126877 (PDF)
Subjects: LCSH: Dimaline, Cherie,
    1975– | LCSH: Monsters in literature. |
    LCSH: Monsters—Symbolic aspects. |
    LCSH: Anxiety in literature. |
    LCSH: Canadian literature—History
    and criticism. | CSH: Indigenous
    literature—History and criticism. |
    LCGFT: Essays.
Classification: LCC PS8607.I53 A82 2023 |
    DDC C814/.6—dc23

First edition, first printing, 2023.
First printed and bound in Canada
by Houghton Boston Printers,
Saskatoon, Saskatchewan.
Copyediting and proofreading by
Joanne Muzak.

All rights reserved. No part of this
publication may be produced, stored
in a retrieval system, or transmitted in
any form or by any means (electronic,
mechanical, photocopying, recording,
or otherwise) without prior written
consent. Contact University of Alberta
Press for further details.

University of Alberta Press supports
copyright. Copyright fuels creativity,
encourages diverse voices, promotes
free speech, and creates a vibrant
culture. Thank you for buying an
authorized edition of this book and for
complying with the copyright laws by
not reproducing, scanning, or distrib-
uting any part of it in any form without
permission. You are supporting writers
and allowing University of Alberta Press
to continue to publish books for every
reader.

The Canadian Literature Centre
acknowledges the support of Dr. Eric
Schloss and the Faculty of Arts for the
CLC Kreisel Lecture delivered by Cherie
Dimaline in April 2022 at the University
of Alberta.

University of Alberta Press gratefully
acknowledges the support received
for its publishing program from
the Government of Canada, the
Canada Council for the Arts, and the
Government of Alberta through the
Alberta Media Fund.

Canada Canada Council Conseil des Arts
        for the Arts   du Canada

Alberta
Government

FOREWORD
THE CLC KREISEL LECTURE SERIES

The CLC Kreisel Lecture Series is an annual event dedicated to nurturing both public and scholarly engagement with the critical concerns of writers in Canada. Each year, an established author is invited to speak about an issue that is important to them, whether because it is close to their heart, foundational to their practice, or a pressing cultural concern; often, it is all these things at once. The series showcases the myriad ways in which writers help us understand the textures of life in this country: it includes lectures about oppression and social justice, cultural identity, place and displacement, the spoils of history, censorship, multilingualism, reading in a digital age, literary history, personal memory, Indigenous resurgence, and the essential function of art. Usually delivered to a live audience on the University of Alberta campus on Treaty 6 Territory and Region 4 of the Métis Nation of Alberta, the Kreisel Lectures frequently also air to audiences across Canada as episodes on CBC Radio's *Ideas*. All of our lectures become books like this one, published in partnership with University of Alberta Press.

Our 2022 lecturer, Cherie Dimaline, is the acclaimed Georgian Bay Métis author of the award-winning YA novel *The Marrow Thieves* (2017), *Empire of Wild* (2019), and *Hunting by Stars* (2021), among other works. As Anna Marie Sewell, amiskwaciwâskahikan / Edmonton writer of Polish and Mi'kmaq descent, noted in her introduction to the lecture, Dimaline is a powerful storyteller who recognizes how important it is for Indigenous youth to see themselves in "stories that matter." Dimaline's work is far reaching, her stories critical for readers of all ages—Indigenous and settler alike. Her literary oeuvre brings together themes of resistance to settler colonialism (including the legacies of Residential Schools and the persistence of colonial structures in the present); climate and ecological crisis; the importance and difficulties of building community; Indigenous resilience and resurgence; place, land, and displacement; and the power of language and storytelling. A deeply personal meditation on the connection between stories and anxiety, her Kreisel Lecture embodies the generosity, humour, and candour that makes her not just a great writer but also a magnanimous human being. Her focus on anxiety struck a chord with the CLC's audience. In the wake of two tumultuous years of pandemic waves and lockdowns, it was, as one audience member put it, "exactly what we all need right now."

The Canadian Literature Centre (CLC) was established in 2006, thanks to the leadership gift of the noted Edmontonian bibliophile Dr. Eric Schloss. In 2007 this lecture series was established in honour of Professor Henry Kreisel. Author, University Professor, and Officer of the Order of Canada, Kreisel was born into a Jewish family in Vienna in 1922. He left his homeland for England in 1938 and was interned in Canada for eighteen months during the Second World War. After studying at the University of Toronto, he was hired in 1947 to teach at the University of Alberta, where he served as Chair of English from 1961 to 1970. He served as Vice-President (Academic) from 1970 to 1975, when he was named University Professor, the highest scholarly award bestowed on its faculty members by the University of Alberta. An inspiring and beloved teacher who taught generations of students to love literature, Professor Kreisel was among the first to champion Canadian literature in university classrooms and to bring the experience of immigrants to modern Canadian literature. As Vice-Provost Florence Glanfield (Indigenous Programming and Research) pointed out in her opening remarks to Dimaline's lecture, Kreisel was also an early ally of Indigenous people, who advocated for Indigenous research and scholarship at the University of Alberta, working hard during his tenure to build relationships between

Indigenous communities and the university. His written works include two novels, *The Rich Man* (1948) and *The Betrayal* (1964), and a collection of short stories, *The Almost Meeting* (1981). His internment diary, alongside critical essays on his writing, appears in *Another Country: Writings by and about Henry Kreisel* (1985). He died in Edmonton in 1991. The generosity and foresight of Professor Kreisel's teaching at the University of Alberta continues to inspire the CLC in its research pursuits, public outreach, and ongoing commitment to the ever-growing richness, complexity, and diversity of writings in Canada.

Sarah Wylie Krotz
Director, Canadian Literature Centre
Edmonton, July 2022

LIMINAIRE

LA COLLECTION DES CONFÉRENCES KREISEL CLC

La série des Conférences Kreisel est un événement annuel consacré à encourager l'engagement du public et des universitaires face aux préoccupations pressentes des écrivains.es au Canada. Chaque année, un.e auteur.e reconnu.e est invité.e à s'exprimer sur un sujet qui lui tient à cœur, que ce soit parce qu'il est à la base de son expérience ou qu'il est urgent et actuel; souvent il s'agit des deux à la fois. La série se compose de conférences sur la résurgence autochtone, l'oppression et la justice sociale, l'identité culturelle, le lieu et le déplacement, les dépouilles de l'histoire, la narration, la censure, la langue, la lecture à l'ère numérique, l'histoire littéraire, la mémoire personnelle, et la nécessité de l'art. Habituellement présentées à un auditoire en direct sur le campus de l'Université de l'Alberta, situé sur le territoire du Traité 6 et de la Région 4 de la Nation Métis, les Conférences Kreisel sont fréquemment diffusées à des auditoires à travers le Canada sous forme d'épisodes diffusés par *Ideas* de la radio CBC. Ces conférences sont également publiées sous forme de livres comme celui-ci, en collaboration avec University of Alberta Press.

Notre conférencière de 2022, Cherie Dimaline, est une auteure métisse de la baie Georgienne, acclamée pour son roman destiné à la jeunesse et primé en 2017, *The Marrow Thieves* et également pour *Empire of Wild* (2019) et *Hunting by Stars* (2021). Comme l'a fait remarquer Anna Marie Sewell, écrivaine d'amiskwaciwâskahikan / Edmonton d'origine polonaise et micmaque, dans son introduction à la conférence, Cherie Dimaline est une conteuse puissante qui reconnaît l'importance pour les jeunes autochtones de s'identifier dans «des histoires qui comptent.»

Son œuvre a une grande portée et ses histoires sont essentielles pour les lecteurs de tous âges, qu'ils soient autochtones ou colons. L'œuvre littéraire de Cherie Dimaline aborde les thèmes de la résistance au colonialisme (y compris l'héritage des pensionnats et la persistance de nos jours de structures coloniales), de la crise climatique et écologique, de l'importance et des difficultés de la construction d'une communauté, de la résilience et de la résurgence autochtones, du lieu, de la terre et du déplacement, ainsi que du pouvoir de la langue et des récits. Telle une méditation profondément personnelle sur le lien entre les histoires et l'anxiété, sa conférence incarne la générosité, l'humour et la franchise qui font d'elle, non seulement, une grande écrivaine, mais aussi un être humain magnanime. L'accent mis par Cherie Dimaline sur l'anxiété a touché une corde sensible dans le public du CLC. Après deux années tumultueuses de pandémie et de confinement, c'était, comme rapporté par un membre du public, «exactement ce dont nous avons tous besoin en ce moment».

Le Centre de littérature canadienne a été créé en 2006 grâce au don directeur de l'illustre bibliophile edmontonien, le docteur Eric Schloss. Cette série de conférences a été créée l'année suivante en l'honneur du professeur Henry Kreisel. Auteur, professeur d'université et Officier de l'Ordre du Canada, celui-ci naît en 1922 à Vienne dans une famille juive. Il quitte son pays natal pour l'Angleterre en 1938 et sera interné au Canada pendant dix-huit mois lors de la Seconde Guerre mondiale. Après ses études à l'Université de Toronto, en 1947 il devient professeur à l'Université de l'Alberta où il dirigera le Département d'anglais de 1961 à 1970. De 1970 à 1975, il est vice-recteur (universitaire), et sera nommé professeur hors rang en 1975, la plus haute distinction scientifique décernée par l'Université de l'Alberta à un membre de son professorat. Professeur hautement respecté, Henry Kreisel inspirera et transmettra l'amour de la littérature à plusieurs générations d'étudiants. Il est un des premiers à défendre la littérature canadienne dans le cadre universitaire et à aborder l'expérience des immigrants au Canada au sein de sa littérature moderne. Comme l'a souligné la vice-rectrice Florence Glanfield (programmation et recherche autochtones) dans ses remarques d'introduction à la conférence de Cherie Dimaline, M. Kreisel a également été un allié de la première heure des peuples autochtones, qui a défendu la recherche autochtone à l'Université de l'Alberta, travaillant dur pendant son mandat pour établir des relations entre les communautés autochtones et l'Université. Son œuvre comprend les romans, *The Rich Man* (1948) et *The Betrayal* (1964), et un recueil de nouvelles intitulé *The Almost Meeting* (1981). Son journal d'internement, accompagné d'articles critiques sur ses écrits, paraît dans *Another Country: Writings by and about Henry Kreisel* (1985). Il est décédé à Edmonton en 1991. Trente plus tard, la générosité et la clairvoyance de l'enseignement du professeur Kreisel à l'Université de l'Alberta continuent d'inspirer le CLC dans ses activités de recherche, sa sensibilisation du public et son engagement envers la richesse, la complexité et la diversité toujours croissantes des écrits au Canada.

Sarah Wylie Krotz
Directrice, Centre de littérature canadienne
Edmonton, juillet 2022

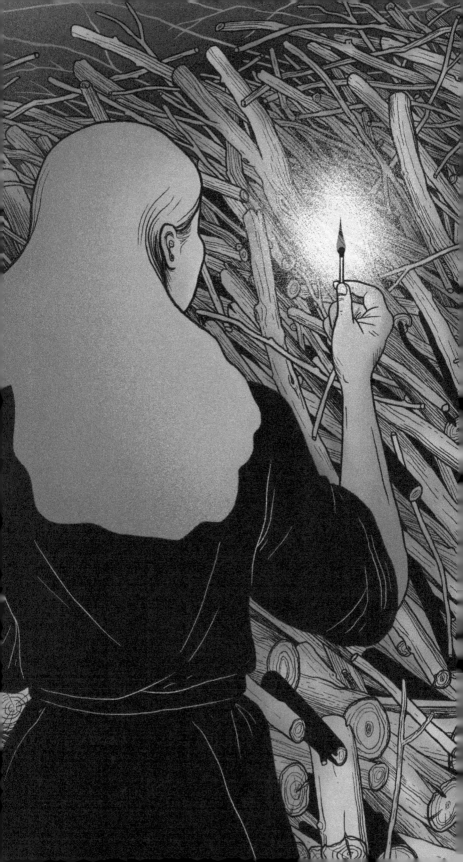

AN ANTHOLOGY OF MONSTERS

HOW STORY SAVES US FROM OUR ANXIETY

For Lee.

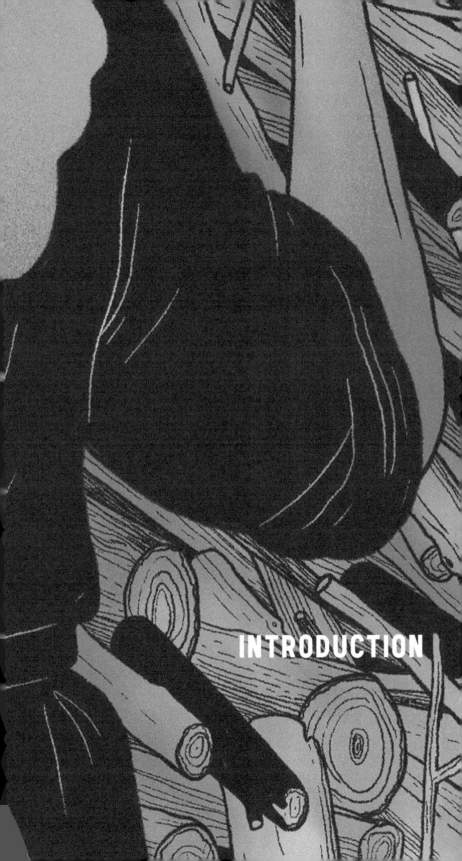

INTRODUCTION

The gift the Kreisel Lecture gives us is the opportunity to come not only as artists, thinkers, and writers, but to come as ourselves. To revel in, as my friend Dr. Florence Glanfield says, "ideas and possibilities." And so, I decided—because of the timeline we are in and because I wanted to come wholly as myself—to talk about the modern monsters that haunt me: anxiety, panic, and all their asshole acquaintances.

I am not a therapist. In fact, I am not trained in any way to treat or even properly handle anxiety and mental wellness. All I have is a lifetime of experience with my own anxiety. All I have to offer are relationships, with myself and my community, with hope and my anxiety, and each one of them I freely hold out. My own personal anxiety has been the mean, twisted, maniacal life partner I drag from apartment to house, and over the midnight mark into every new year, despite promises to finally kick it to the curb. It sticks and it sings and, more than anything, it tells stories. So, if there is something here you can take, then you are welcome to it.

The good news, in spite of the lack of professional under- standing or the ability to give you easy self-help guidance, is that I have been taught to tell my own stories. And so, anxiety and I, with our storytelling genes, we exist in a kind of friendly/ dysfunctional competition that's been set up between us—who can tell the most powerful stories and which one will determine how I feel that day. The scoreboard changes all the time and I am not always winning, but I am, at least, in the running.

Basically, this is the story of a lifelong dance with anxiety and how story can help reshape the ways in which we think, the ways we cope, and the very choreography of that dance. What I want to talk about is how our anxiety uses stories against us, how we can create stories to fight back, and how life is basically an anthology of both. And, most importantly, that it is normal and okay for both to exist at the same time.

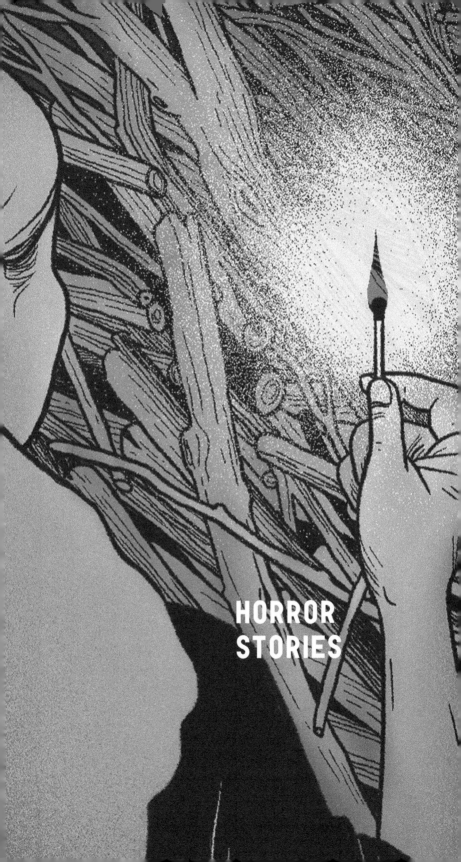

HORROR
STORIES

IN THE BEGINNING

I imagine that the first time norepinephrine flooded into my body, causing my heart to race, my skin to sweat, my mind to spin, was when I was born. There's no way to prove this, no way to untap the memory of the rush of light and sound as I entered into the world and a subsequent release of adrenaline. But I can imagine it. I can imagine it in full colour and detail because this is what my brain likes to do—loves to do—imagine worst-case scenarios, especially as they pertain to me. Maybe my first cry in the delivery room was the standard infant bewilderment and discomfort, but maybe also it was the tingly sensation of chemical fear pouring into newly unfurling limbs. That would be very like me, very Cherie, to take this monumental, almost celestial moment and render it in shades of red emergency and dark panic.

What I do know for sure is the day I remember having my first actual panic attack. I was seven and it was the day of my First Communion (probably a sign that my relationship with the Catholic Church wasn't going to work out). I was wearing what my mother insisted was "an adorable" knee-length white dress with a matching straw hat, set at a jaunty angle. After all, it was 1982 and I needed to make sure my feathered bangs were visible. I was already worried since everyone else was wearing floor-length dresses and veils, very bridal (which I thought was also very cultish, but who was I to judge 1980s Christian couture?). My friends thought my choice was bold, even a bit risqué. Really, I had left the entire decision to my mother, who, with her permed mullet and tinted glasses, made the fashion choices in the house.

Just before we left for the church, I started to get nervous. I was supposed to "eat something" so that I wouldn't interrupt the afternoon's events with requests for a Happy Meal, but I couldn't seem to get anything into my stomach. Chewing was too much stimulation. My gut did not want to be interrupted from the knots it was busy tying. I thought, "What if I mess up?" And because I've always had a pretty active imagination, I had scenarios of the ways in which I could mess up.

What if I pee my pants in front of everyone?

What if I say the wrong words and the priest stops the whole thing to demand I find the right ones?

What if I take in the Eucharist and then throw up the Eucharist, full exorcist-style? Which would be the worst case of bad timing in the history of the world.

None of this was very likely, but there was this voice, this tiny hiss from somewhere in the back of my brain that asked, *But what if it does happen? Just, really, think about it—what if?* So, I did. I thought about each scenario. And as I did, the voice got louder, from the middle of my head, *That's it, you're doing the right thing. Remember, prepare for the worst...*

Then, my mind was galloping, going over each nightmare situation in full colour, with guest stars even and an impressive soundtrack. That's when the pins and needles showed up, starting in my knees and moving into my butt. The voice in my head was confident now, even chatty. *You wouldn't be so worried if you didn't believe this could happen, which means, it will happen.*

I remember how the dimensions of my living room suddenly changed. This was the early '80s so it was basically macrame and orange furniture. And everything got brighter and it was as if I was looking down a cardboard tube, the way I did with rolls of wrapping paper before my brother and I beat the shit out of each other with them. And then the voice suggested, just a suggestion, no big deal, *Psssst. Maybe you're dying.*

And then I was. I was very clearly dying, there was no other way to adequately describe the feeling. It was a kind of knowing, a certainty that the worst had arrived. I moved carefully to the bathroom and closed the door. I didn't want to worry my parents. I didn't want my grandmother to have to watch me die in my risqué white communion dress. And I sat on the floor, because the tiles were cold and I could make myself real small, and I tried to remember how to breathe. And then, there was a knock at the door telling me to hurry up, it was time to go.

How could I go? How could I do anything? And then I realized, how could I not? What would I say to get out of this event? And what would that then mean for my eternal Catholic soul? I was still young enough to feel like there were some things I had no say in, even if it had to do with me.

So I tried to rein in this terrible thing, this feeling of intimate doom. I breathed deeply, forcing my lungs to open. I swallowed spit, forcing my mouth to work. I crawled to my hands and knees, then consciously requested the co-operation of each muscle in standing. And then, I opened the door, waiting for the looks on my family's faces, the horror, the fear, when they saw that I was indeed dying, right in front of them...

And nobody said anything, nobody asked me if I was okay. Nobody screamed with horror at my appearance or called 911. In fact, nobody really noticed anything other than my leotards had to be straightened a bit. Which then meant, I must look the same. That there were no outward indications of that fact that I was very clearly experiencing the end of the world. What was going on?

Not to worry, the voice had an answer, and now it was speaking from the front of my brain, like, in the driver's seat. *Ooooh, you're not dying. You're just going crazy.*

And then I went to the church to take my first communion in front of two hundred people. And while I might have otherwise forgotten it, that day was sharply carved into my memory.

Once the capacity for panic had hollowed out a comfortable space, it visited often. And then, here's the kicker, I spent time every single day worrying about whether or not I would have another "episode," which, if you're familiar with the phenomenon of a panic attack, does NOT help one bit.

I didn't know what it was, I didn't have a name for it. No one I knew had ever said the word *anxiety*, and mental health was still a topic that people didn't openly talk about, so I thought it was truly me losing my mind. Which meant, if I wanted to be normal, if I wanted to be okay, I had to keep it hidden. And it terrified me.

From that day on, I held this fracturing fear in my tiny ribcage. It made me shy. It made me prone to fistfights. It made me ashamed. I got used to keeping secrets, which meant I started to keep secrets I shouldn't, secrets others swore me to. I silenced myself in case, when I opened my mouth, I screamed instead of whispering. I started craving patterns, counting things and moving certain ways, because if I could control the patterns, then maybe I could make myself safe with that tightly orchestrated control.

LOOKING FOR SOLACE

In search of control, but also being the kind of kid I was—one with a voracious appetite for story and adventure—I became an avid reader. Reading was the world distilled onto paper, which meant I could handle it. Which meant I could experience life from a place of safety. These literary worlds became the places I returned to again and again looking for some kind of solace.

I read everything I could find, everything there was. But not once, until I stumbled on to French existentialists and the Beat poets as a preteen (I think it's a requirement of turning fourteen), did I ever even imagine that others were experiencing the terror of carrying a well-oxygenated fire inside your bones, so close to your lungs that it could stop you from breathing. And even then, it wasn't until my early twenties, when I found stories that more closely resembled my own, that I finally read about anxiety and understood just who the voice was that I had been speaking to all these years (that's a lie, I didn't speak to the voice, it just kind of spoke AT me, all judgey and passive aggressive). It was anxiety and it was not mine alone. Instead, I found, I belonged to this silent club that kept anxiety's secrets and tended to its every whim.

But what if I had read those stories earlier? What if I had read about a girl, maybe even a halfbreed girl from the Georgian Bay who could throw a mean right hook, who lived with panic instead of dreams? I just finished a manuscript for that girl. It's called *Funeral Songs for Dying Girls* (Penguin, 2023). This is the opening of that story:

> There's a film company whose logo comes on
> before the movie starts. It's a boy sitting in a
> crescent moon, fishing the sky. That's the closest

thing I can think of to explain how I feel in the attic, sitting at the window watching the fog roll, or the leaves fall, or the snow chase itself around gravestones in the cemetery below. I feel like a boy with a fishing pole and a shitty sense of hunt.

What could you possibly pull out of the heavens to eat? What kind of bait would you use to hook a star? Some old people say stars were people once. So maybe you could find your ancestors out there, and yank grannies out of the dark like slick trout.

My room is like my brain—kind of messy, full of too much, organized in ways only I can decipher. And then there's the way my brain has bled the need for patterns into its space. So now I do math with the digital numbers on my alarm clock (12:34—1+2=3 + 1 more number=4) and symmetry has become increasingly important. (I touch the tips of each big toe twice on the hardwood before I pull them into my hammock at night.)

I wanted to ask Dad about the patterns. I wanted to know if maybe my mother counted too much or that when she scratched her left ear, if maybe she buzzed angrily beneath her skin until she scratched her right one, with the same amount of pressure. It's probably one of those conversations that would get cut short where, instead of speaking, he just pulled at his beard and slowly leaned back until he felt safely removed from my quiet hysteria.

I think a lot about the lack of literature I had to rely on back then, about looking for some resemblance of what I was feeling, what I was dealing with, in the world. There were no characters who counted seconds before they moved to make sure their existence was measured and balanced. There were no stories about the fear of being alone in the moments before sleep, a prime opening slot for the terror to seep in. And I think about the kids who could end up on their own bathroom floor wondering if they are dying. I think that there is a real responsibility, and also a real joy, in building a room in our collective house— a room for scared children who think they are all alone with their fire. We, survivors of anxiety experienced at a young age, need to work to build the safe room where these kids can feel okay, and maybe even come to understand that they are not alone.

NIGHT TERRORS

Here's an example of a pretty common Horror Story that I am sure we can all relate to. And if you can't relate to it, you need to write a book about it because, congratulations, you are a unicorn.

It's 2 a.m. I have been in bed for an hour, wondering if I've watched enough intellectually stunted television on Netflix to have lulled my brain into thinking "hey, there are no thoughts left tonight" so that I can safely put my laptop away and actually sleep. So I do it, I close the computer and set it on the nightstand and hope that I don't have to open it again. That's the trick, getting through this step quick enough that I don't start the spiral down into what-ifs, and slow enough that I don't jolt my body into thinking there is more to do. Everything is about timing at this point. Especially: don't think about time. If you do, you'll count the hours you have until you need to be functioning—meetings, work left undone, a to-do list—no, don't think of the to-do list! Lists needs to be checked off or they are testaments to failure, especially in the middle of the night when you can't do much about them. When you're up and doing things, they help keep you on track. But when you're in bed, they are a numbered letter you've written to your future self about how much she is already lacking, already behind.

But let's say, I've done it—I am numb and tired and I really could sleep, so I close my eyes. Holy shit, my eyes are closed! And then there are the few seconds before my head grabs a narrative and takes me into sleep. Okay, I am thinking about a house I want to build in some great future where I've made enough money to build a house. The living room will look like a curiosity shop. The wallpaper will be something ridiculous— maybe smoking nuns or pink monkeys—and then the doorbell rings and I open it and there's anxiety. Before I can slam it shut it says, *Hey girl, remember in 2012 when you were at the airport in Montreal and the Air Canada employee at the desk said, "Have a great flight" and you said, "You too"?*

And that stops me, now I can't shut the door. Anxiety lets itself in, sits on the chair, and really leans in: *Oh, and remember there was that party you went to in your early twenties, when they were giving out free Jägermeister and you were still broke enough to think you needed to drink the hell out of that Jägermeister because, well, it was free, and then you got so drunk you started an argument with that group of strangers who said you were an idiot? Oh man, you really were an idiot. Wait...let me play that back in detail for you...*

And my eyes are open and I am trapped in my small and numerous humiliations, things I had pushed aside because they were tiny and I needed to live, things so insignificant that they didn't bare remembering. But anxiety, she remembers. She remembers the weather and what I wore and the looks on people's faces, even people I never saw again, people who probably have no memory of me or what I said when I decided a party was a good place to take a political stand about whatever the hell I made a political stand about. And anxiety makes me feel this kind of twisted guilt, as if this discomfort I feel in the remembering of these small things is also somehow an indication that I deserve to feel them, that I have committed wrongs.

I have the horrifying talent of still feeling embarrassed about something I said or did twenty years ago. Do I remember how I felt when I was on the front page of the *New York Times* Arts section? No. But I remember, word for word, a mean tweet directed at me from a man who had never met me but decided to question everything about me as if I was not a real person. Do I remember the joy I experienced when I first got on the bestsellers list? A bit, it was great. But what I remember in vivid detail is how I felt when someone replied to my author photo that accompanied the news online with "Sounds boring, nice tits though."

Let's forget about others for a second. Why are we so mean to ourselves? What is it about anxiety that makes us so full of empathy and understanding for others but so decidedly evil to ourselves?

MANIFESTING GOOD AND
THE GOOD DAYS AS BAD OMENS

There is a school of thought that says "what you focus on is what grows." On the surface, this is a lovely sentiment. It says that we are responsible for our own success, that we should put all our energy into what it is we want to accomplish or achieve or receive. This kind of "law of attraction" philosophy has been designed, as far as I can tell, to let us feel empowered, and it is a great way to encourage positive thinking, getting people to focus on the things they can change, to not get mired in the bullshit that can drag you down.

The problem is, for someone with anxiety who can't help but focus all their energy and time on the horrible things that have happened or that may happen in the future, it says "YOU ARE GUARANTEEING DISASTER!" It's a crippling idea, reinforced by a theory that was meant to empower. And I'm not saying I disagree with the sentiment that we should keep our goals at the centre of our thoughts. In fact, I work hard to this day to "focus" on the positive, to try to give as much energy and time as I can to those bright, beautiful things that I want to see manifest. But at the same time, I am weighted by a new guilt, that I might be the one making things difficult for myself, which, in turn, only makes things more difficult for the people who love me.

Some moments catch you really off guard. Some days, you find yourself laughing or smiling or even just sinking into the comfort of a chair in the middle of the afternoon with nothing on your mind and suddenly you realize, *I'm not anxious. What the hell am I doing? Why am I okay? Why am I happy?* It's unusual. It's suspect. And then, that reprieve is gone. Replaced by the familiar sting of invisible catastrophe—and somehow, that feels better. Your body knows how to settle into those movements. This is the known, and with it comes some kind of painful comfort.

And it's not just that "the devil you know" kind of thinking; instead, it's more of that old fear thinking: *disaster is always worse if it catches you unaware, and you, my friend, are blissfully unaware.* The higher the height you fall from, the more devastating the impact. So when put this way (and this is how the anxious mind puts it), being happy is just inviting disaster, asking for trouble, and, in fact, an invitation to be pushed off an edge.

Here's how a person (i.e., me) could end up feeling conflicted about good news or success. If something good happens, that means in the cosmic sense of it all—also according to old wives everywhere—the other shoe has to drop, the opposite and terrifying other shoe. And of course, it must drop for two reasons: one, all things comes in pairs (remember those comforting patterns? Ha!); and two, the other shoe is too heavy not to drop. No universe could possibly hold it up forever. The reason it feels so heavy is because the other shoe is full of anxiety, and I have given it so much weight, a lifetime of weight. This is how I allow anxiety to ruin even the best things.

So one day I decided, fate has one foot. I don't know, maybe it had diabetes at some point. Maybe there was an accident of some sort. Or better yet, fate is like those old timey ghosts that they draw with one long tendril as the bottom half of their body in cartoons. But I'm calling it: fate has one foot and therefore only requires one shoe. So when that thing drops, whatever that good, great thing might be, that's it. There is nothing coming after it. It is not fated. It is not a given. If another shoe wants to drop, then that ghost is going to have to float home and get a new one.

We need to remind ourselves that something terrible isn't going to happen every time something good happens. And anyway, why do we think that good needs to be balanced with bad? Maybe instead we reframe it as "loud happiness" is balanced by "quiet calm"? Maybe the counter balance to say, a big award is just solitary gratitude?

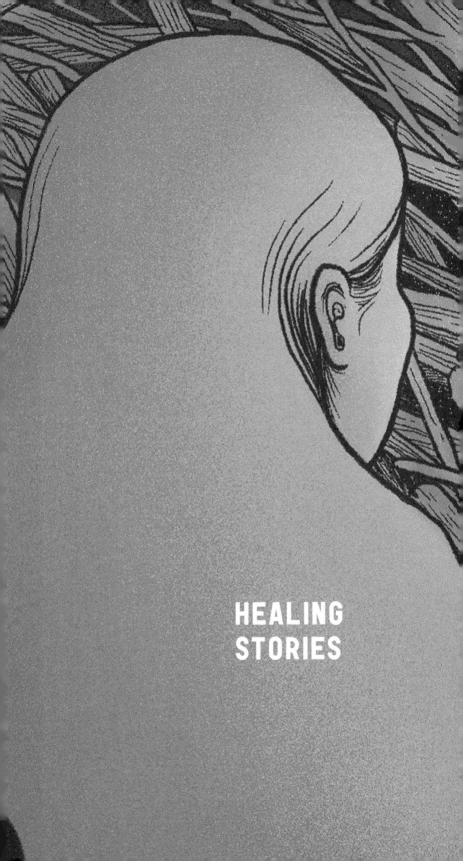

HEALING
STORIES

I was lucky enough to grow up in a house full of stories. My mother's family—both on her mother's and father's sides—are Georgian Bay Métis and are all storytellers, which, for some of them, just means real fancy liars. Especially since they hunt and fish—there's always a story blown out of proportion.

Last year, during a particularly bad month of anxiety, I spoke with an Elder in Saskatchewan who advised me to do two things: first, see a doctor if I hadn't already (I had—I would never not advise anyone with anxiety to take whatever route works for them). And second, to write the story of my specific community, that it would have the ability and the language to make me feel better. She reminded me that the one defence I've always had against anxiety, the one defence my family and ancestors employed to try to keep us safe, was still readily available to me: story.

So I sat down and wrote out everything I could about my eccentric and amazing community—not the statistics, not the historical halfbreed petitions, or the court cases for rights, but the wider and also smaller story *of us* and how it relates to *my* particular story. I wrote out the stories and places and language of my own small/huge family. And getting it down on paper, I had to take time to think about each grandmother, to remember the way they always said "*the* Jesus" or put "you" at the end of a sentence as emphasis, like this: "You come back on time, you."

I wrote about who I am descended from, where my stories come from, and everything I could remember that I had ever been told. It turns out, the Elder was right (I admit, she usually is)—this story was absolute medicine. This story reminded me, continues to remind me, that I am a part of something bigger, an important part of a larger narrative. It's a story that I return to in moments when I am feeling too small, too mixed, too colonized. It has become like a worry doll or a smooth rock to rub—that I am of these specific and resilient people, all the way back in time rolling up to today. It tells me in no uncertain terms that I am enough.

There are all kinds of stories, and the stories I grew up with, had different purposes.

MAPPING AND KINSHIP

Before my family's genealogy was carefully drawn up for the membership work my nation's government was carrying out, I already knew that my grandfather's family had come from the Red River and also from Anishnaabe Territory; that my Mère's— my grandmother's—family came from Anishnaabe and French halfbreed families around the Great Lakes and that I had relatives on Manitoulin Island because one of the families had split between the Georgian Bay mainland and the island. I knew this because these movements were mapped out in stories that were handed down to me.

MEDICINE

These stories are not metaphorical by nature, but could often veer in that direction if the situation required it. They were a part of the long walks my grandmother and her sisters Flora and Ethel took me on to pick plants in the ditches by the road and in the fields that didn't belong to us. They were the remedies I was subjected to as a child when arguing that all I needed was a Flintstone vitamin, for cripes' sake. Things like plantain for rashes, tobacco smoke for earaches, spit for mosquito bites and blood stains, onions for fever, Easter Sunday water for syrups, and pine oil for salves. I have a cabinet in my home now that, over the years, has gathered mason jars with homemade labels and the tools of the trade—I suppose it was inevitable that my own children would receive this kind of home-brewed medicine—bear grease for skin conditions, rat root to keep sickness at bay. (Don't worry, they've also gotten Flintstone vitamins, as well.)

LAUGHTER AND SURVIVAL

These were the stories that we reveled in, the ones that got told the most, the loudest, and on repeat. They recounted exploits, made legends out of men, and reminded us that no matter what, laughter is the biggest sound, the one that clears the space for all the other work that needs dedicated room to bloom. These stories reminded me that I was lucky to be born into my family, that I was blessed to be a part of my community. And this is important, because family can piss you off real quick and real often, so it's good to remember that love and gratitude. It's good to feel magic and wonder creeping around the edges of the gridlines that lay out modern life. These stories continue to show me that the unknown is not always something we should seek to control, to figure out and nail down, that uncertainty does not always mean doom or chaos. That sometimes the unknown is so beautiful as to hold us when we need it, to provide joy and escape, or knowledge and grounding.

WARNINGS

These stories were often scary, sometimes unbelievable, but always told as if they had just happened and could be backed up by several eyewitnesses. They were the Shadow Men walking into yards, possession of children by things as innocuous as a toad, vengeful animals who played dead until an opportune moment, how quickly you could drown in the bay (accompanied by a side story on how to find those bodies the lake claimed), and then, of course, there was the story that captured my imagination: The Rougarou.

The Rougarou features in my stories but by no means did I create him. In many ways, the Rougarou helped to create me. If you have not heard of him and have not read *Empire of Wild* or any of the great Rougarou stories told across the homeland, let me give you a quick Rougarou 101.

ROUGAROU

The Rougarou is a creature who lives in Métis communities and also in some Cajun settlements. In Louisiana, they even have an annual Rougarou Festival. He is a wolf- or dog-like entity that usually walks and talks like a man. Every community, every storyteller has a different way of interpreting him and the specifics about him—sometimes he is charming and charismatic, sometimes he is terrifying and vicious. In some stories he wears a suit and moccasins, in others he has only his fur and is more animal than human. There are stories about him in my community. One was made into a play in the 1950s, written by the local priest, about how Rougarou brought together the First Nations, Métis, and French settlers in the area to hunt him, which he allowed as long as it meant they would finally learn how to work together. My Mère swears she met him in the field going to get her water one day. In her story, she stood very still, bucket and wooden spoon in hand, and watched as the creature woke, turned back into the local priest and ran away into the woods, presumably headed back to the church. (This story makes me wonder if the play version of the benevolent creature bringing the people together was just the Rougarou coming up with some good PR for himself.)

In many stories, his ultimate role is revealed—to teach and protect the community, even if his ways are harsh. In my Great Auntie's kitchen, we learned that there were several ways a person who identified as male could become a Rougarou—among them, breaking Lent, lying, being violent to another person (especially a partner), and overhunting (or overfishing). So Rougarou stories were used as a kind of warning story for how to behave in a way that was community acceptable. For myself, growing up as a girl, the stories were used to keep me safe, especially from men. I learned that walking along the road, particularly during summer would leave me vulnerable to Rougarou attacks (we live in cottage country so the summers meant an influx of strangers), that we were to always travel in packs and stick to the well-lighted areas. As we got older, we were warned not to pick a partner who exhibited any of the traits that could mean that one day we would wake up with a wolf in the bed.

What my grandmother and her sisters were telling me in a way that you could tell a child was the grim reality that women in our community were regularly assaulted, and experienced domestic abuse and violence. Putting all that history and horror into a story meant I listened, I took care to follow the rules that would keep me safer (in theory), and that I could also hold it at a distance as a story, so not have it take up space in my life as a weight. They were trying to use story to hold anxiety in place and not let it run amok as I grew up.

In this way, story was used as a way to deter anxiety while still doing the necessary work of invoking the desired feelings and behaviours. These stories were also a way for the old women to get their point across without being ignored by their listeners. We took them seriously but we also enjoyed the thrill of being scared while remaining safe without their reach.

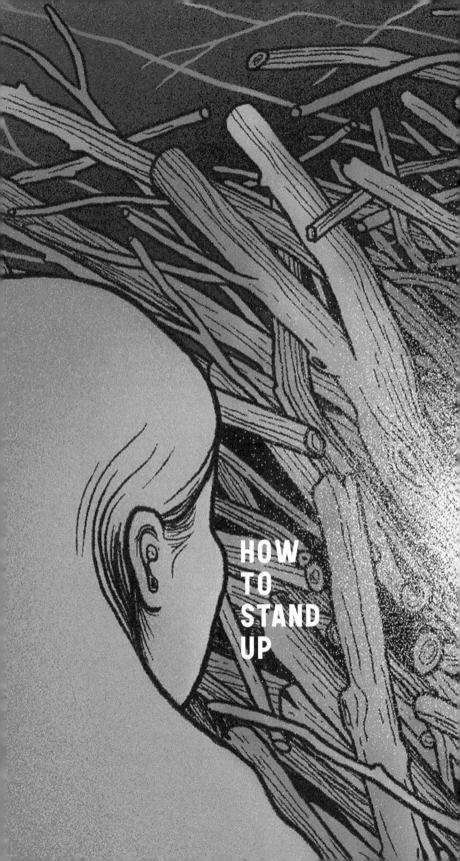

HOW
TO
STAND
UP

LEE MARACLE AND THE WAY TO STAND

My late mentor, great friend, and profound teacher Lee Maracle, one of our greatest storytellers, had no time for anxiety. Being around her was a marvel. She forgave herself everything. It was beautiful to see. She thought about things, ruminated on them, and then let go of the negativity that wasn't going to do her anything but harm. Just...poof...let it go.

I remember in great detail, the feeling I had on the day she and I finished editing my first book. It had been a dream to work with her, literally a dream come true, and also one of the hardest things I've ever had to do. Being vulnerable in front of one of your heroes is not an easy thing. And at that point in my life, anxiety had taken the breath from my body and I couldn't even read my own words aloud. It's hard to form words when you are gasping for air. And Lee saw this without me pointing it out, without her pointing it out. Her response was not to coddle, but to help me break through. She would make me stand in the hallway of the university where she had an office and read my work, loud and sure, no matter how many people were walking by or gathered at the computers set up just outside her room.

"You have to stand for your words," she would tell me. And when that wasn't enough, she made an association that ensured I would have to be confident, invoking the one thing that could make me act without thought of myself or my anxiety.

"I can hear your grandmother in your work. So you stand for your grandmother," she said. And I did. It was months of her teaching me not just how to be a better writer, but how to be the kind of writer who could write with conviction, with change in mind, and to weather whatever storms that conviction would inevitably attract. Because, she explained, when you write with both truth and love, refusing to shirk away from the hard stuff, there is always going to be a response that is equally cutting and constructive at the same time.

The day we finished that manuscript, I felt buoyant, like everything was going to be different and that I had earned the right to walk across that level ground of my story-scape because I was the one who had levelled it. Lee was good at that—doing so much work and then heaping praise on the smallest steps you took in taking on the slightest of burdens, especially when she could see how hard the approach to even begin was.

Her office was just north of Chinatown in Toronto, so I walked down Spadina Road and went into the first shop I found. I picked up a tiny charm with a rabbit on it, the kind of thing you put on a keyring, and bought it. Then I stood outside—it was grey and windy—and held that little plastic charm and really felt exactly how I felt at that moment. Every bit of it. And I still have that charm. And every time I hold it, I am brought right back to that moment. Right back to that feeling. I try to do that more, nowadays. I try to feel all the beauty and power when it comes. We deserve it all. We deserve to have what Lee called "full banquet living."

Lee once said something that has allowed me to truly understand that walls can come down, roadblocks are temporary, and everything can be celebrated. She said, "My life has been a long, slow journey over very sharp rocks, but goddamn it if I didn't dance over every last one of them."

I continue to spend my life learning the choreography that will carry me over the sharp rocks, that will bring me to the water's edge, that will always bring me home. And that means finding the ways to celebrate and live fully even when the world around me seems inhospitable and my anxiety tries to cover my eyes so the way is hard to see. Lee reminds me—reminds all of us—that we don't need to see the path to know that we are on it. We need to trust ourselves and those who came before us to break that path, like she did for so many of us.

THE DOUBLE-EDGED SWORD OF BEING A WRITER

From the story about my First Communion/First Panic Attack, you can clearly see how being a writer, a creator of stories, could make things worse. Like all artists, I have a really muscular imagination. That means, I am a goddamn maestro at coming up with worst-case scenarios. To this day, I feel like I need to stay awake as a passenger on road trips so that I can focus to make sure we don't get into a car accident. (I have no idea how this makes sense, but anxiety is rarely logical.)

Being an author also means that you are working with and from your own personal feelings, experiences, and points of view. Real intimate stuff. For someone who can't bear to even begin to think about being judged, maybe having a job where your work is regularly and publicly critically reviewed is not the best decision.

But why is judgement so hard? Why do we care what others think so much? Why is Twitter the worst thing to happen to anxious people since cellphones?

Maybe because there is nothing anyone could say about us that we haven't already said to ourselves. The one sliver of hope in all the negative self-talk is that we can work to push it away by saying "they're just thoughts, not reality" and remind ourselves that its part of the whole anxiety game. So, for example, I, like many creatives, have experienced and continue to, at times, experience imposter syndrome. *I don't deserve this, that was a fluke, I am not actually a good writer.* Now, if I go on Twitter and someone says, "that book was a fluke, she's not actually a good writer," then it hits like a truth, like a memory, because I've thought about it so much that, even if I manage to dismiss it, it has left an imprint. And so maybe they're right! Maybe I was right to question myself! And if that's true, then what else is true?! You can see the wheels picking up speed...

LIVING THROUGH WRITING

The good thing about being a writer, and the reason I always advise people to write things out, is that you get to organize yourself, figure out how you feel, and record the truth before your anxiety twists everything like a funhouse mirror. Think about how much better you feel when you take all the dangling threads of deadlines and errands and put them into a list—then you know what you have to do and for who and for when. You have something to refer to, so you don't have to keep every all the information untangled in your head alone. (Disclaimer from above: do not think of the list at night when you're trying to sleep!)

I always loved the diaries of Anaïs Nin, the prolific early twentieth-century French diarist and writer. She wrote everything—her entire life down to the minute. She said once that she only truly lived her life when she was writing it, as if the experiences were recorded while she was moving through but that she lived inside of them when she wrote about them. This made a lot of sense to me.

One of my favourite things about writing is not world building; instead, it's world examination. When I'm writing, I can change the cadence and volume to whatever I need it to be in order to really understand, to live in a moment. I am so much braver when I write. Things make sense. I can take on the hard stuff and also have an opportunity to see the good things. This is why it's important to write about the good, the great, the beautiful as much as you write about the horrific or frustrating—to have a record of both. *The Marrow Thieves* was a book that was written from both ends of that spectrum.

The first draft of *Thieves* was written in six weeks. It was when the national conversation on Residential Schools really picked up. I had read this article in the paper that asked Canada if they really thought it was genocide, like a literal poll. A poll about children, about grandparents. As if it was something up for debate. I was angry. I wanted to find a way to capture that terror, to bring home the people forced down to mere statistics, to personalize the horror for a wider group, maybe even the whole country, the way it was deeply personal for so many. That is where the first draft came from. But then, I had to go back in. Because I wanted the book to be for our youth first and foremost—a way to give them hope and make them proud. I wanted them to know that they were the absolute answer, all our hope. I wanted to explain that even at the end of the world, there are still worlds worth fighting for and that, as Indigenous people, we had an intimate knowledge of how to fight in a way that ensured we didn't lose ourselves. So I went back in with that in mind—all the strength, all the beauty, all the good fight. And I rewrote the book, over and over, until both were true—the abject horror of the schools and a world where such a thing could happen, and the hope and beauty of a people who could survive it, who could laugh the loudest, love the hardest.

Writing that book changed my life. It was also a story that needed me to stand for it, all over the world, in several languages, and years later, I am still standing. Lee made sure I could do that. She gave me perspective, so that I remember that we have a responsibility to represent those who came before us and to be there for those who will come after, to always stand for our stories, which is something so much bigger than a monster under the bed.

CREATING OPTIMISM

In the spring of 2022, I had just finished a manuscript (*Ven.Co*, Random House Canada, HarperCollins US, 2023) about what, on the surface, is a coven trying to come together in the face of violence and oppression to tear down the patriarchy. Added to this "Hex the Patriarchy" theme is remembering that we have never been disconnected from the ground (our roots) and the sky (a personal connection with the divine) no matter what anyone has tried to convince us. I started writing it during the pandemic when we were all feeling suspended in the ether, like someone had hit the pause button and the only things getting through were sharp and scary. I could write the book because I had spent years trying to remind myself that I am not powerless, that I am not separate and alone and at the whim of others. That there was still magic left in the world and as someone who felt every-thing deeply—every tone, every change, every whisper—that that meant I would also be one of the people who could feel that magic. I also wanted to acknowledge how hard it is to take all that in when you're busy being distracted by the sharp and scary. This is from the opening, when the protagonist is walking home, preoccupied by worries:

> The moon watched Lucky cut a small figure down the grey sidewalk, giving her a half wink from between the streetcar wires and eternity. Eyes on her Converse and the asphalt, she missed the moon and she missed the tall woman in a salmon pink tulle gown skipping into an alley ahead of her. When Lucky crossed the street to avoid two drunks fighting, she also missed the two foxes carrying a netted bag of oranges between them. She didn't see a half dozen bats careening from an

open apartment window, looping calligraphy onto the dark sky then chasing one another into the parkette. Focused inward and down, she missed all the magic and chance.

Dread, Lucky kept thinking. Nothing ever happens except more of the same.

KEEPING
AN
ANTHOLOGY

(OF BOTH,
BUT
IN ORDER)

HOW TO AVOID THE EDIT REEL

I'm pretty good at pep talks, especially when it comes to building myself up in the moments I need to, which sometimes means every morning. I know exactly what I need to hear and the ways in which I will best hear it. *You've earned this, years of community effort, decades of hard work, this moment is nothing compared to what you've done to be able to walk in that door,* etc.

But now imagine what I could do if we put that effort in reverse—if I was instead giving myself a dressing-down, of sorts? *Who exactly are you that you think you deserve this? At best you're skilled at convincing yourself and others that you are someone. But who are you really? What makes you think you deserve this happiness? Do you think you're better than others?* etc.

Except add to the negative words, high-def video. Like, a top of the line, professional-grade finely produced audiovisual presentation—so adept, so sharp, that you can feel the cold and smell the fire when they flash across the screen. This, friends, is the dreaded Edit Reel. The PowerPoint of doom. The out-of-context, flashing, screaming reel of shame that cuts out all the steps and just reminds you of the fall, as if all you did was fall.

The Edit Reel is a torture chamber. It's where we take ourselves to be punished. It's where all the what-ifs go to sing karaoke together—loud and screechy. It's where our worst fears and most shameful moments meet up and sing duets, without context and free from reason. Of course, reflection is an important tool to grow, to change, to become better versions of ourselves. But when we start to live completely in that realm—reflection without perspective—then it becomes a problem. Likewise, if we try to cut scenes whole-cloth. Here's one example from my very naïve and very young years.

Early on, I made the mistake of thinking perfection was an actual real thing, and more so, that it was an actual, real thing I could achieve. I thought that maybe if I was perfect, I wouldn't be anxious anymore. So I would do this thing, where I tried to "reset." I would clean my room, set up my books and belongings in aesthetically pleasing ways, and then start again. I was basically trying to live an Instagram life before Instagram existed. Which we all know is absolutely impossible. I put myself under New Year's resolution–style pressure every day, all in hopes of not being anxious anymore. (If it wasn't already a cliché, this would be the exact moment in history when the phrase "adding fuel to the fire" would have been invented.)

What I thought was, I needed to remove all of the stress, cut out every moment that wasn't joy, to have a life story that wasn't tragic. The only way to prevent more stress was to remove every second of it from my existence. Now, obviously I was very young and optimistic, thinking that all the shiny, happy people I saw on TV and at dinner parties were living without even the knowledge that a monster *could* live under your bed. What I came to realize, after about a thousand "resets" that never lasted more than an hour, was that I needed to find a way to safely carry that anxiety so that it wasn't the entirety of my story. I needed to learn how to curate an anthology.

HOW TO CURATE THE ANTHOLOGY

So then, how do we do it? How do we hold both the terror and
the joy? How do we carry this fire in our ribs so close to the
pages of greatness without burning it all to the ground? For me,
it's about managing the tone. I try to dial the joy all the way up.
These stories are full-colour. And the more difficult stuff? The
stories that hurt? I render these in sepia, pale and light, so that
they don't jump out at me when I try to flip through this collection of stories that make up my life. They exist, they have a place,
but they are not everything. I will not frame them as such.

So first things first: we accept that life is, as Lee pointed
out, full banquet living, that there are sharp rocks but that we
can choreograph joy and accomplishment over their edges. And
then we make sure that the difficult parts don't take up the most
pages—that there is balance. That we remember to celebrate
ourselves as much as we criticize.

All of my characters have a little bit of me in them. That's
no secret, it's what we do as writers: we mine, we borrow, we
obsess. So all of my characters are a bit anxious. The great news
is that that then gives me the opportunity to give them reprieve,
which then gives me reprieve. I work through my own issues by
working through theirs. It's a bit like playing god, but without
all the extra work of world creating and prayer answering. It's
through this process that I find peace with who I am, how I
think, the ways in which I live. Here is Lucky from the book
mentioned earlier, realizing that what sets her apart also allows
her access to a great and full world:

> The sun was high over the Quarter. The buildings
> here were narrow and low. Where they did have
> second or third floors, each one was wrapped in

iron filigree balconies like cursive writing. Across the street, between two slim buildings, a wooden gate had been left opened and she saw a path there that opened into a small, lush garden, with green ferns and a crooked palm tree and a small stone fountain. She wondered if every place in New Orleans had a secret garden, if every place was so witchy and beautiful. And for the first time, she was filled with an enormous pride for who she was—what she was, all of it. That pride filled the spaces between her bones so that it was impossible not to stand tall.

Anxiety makes everything feel very big or very small, depending on which is more hurtful to you in the moment. Being suddenly relieved of anxiety in this moment gave her a clear understanding that this was the life she had been running towards. Not necessarily New Orleans, not a distant dot on a map, not a brand-new career, but a life full of secret gardens.

When I was little, I was obsessed with *The Secret Garden*. Not the asshole protagonist who from page one has some pretty asshole views on India and her "servants." But rather the idea that a world could exist behind a grief-built wall. That there are still places full of magic. It's also why we collectively as a society fell in love with the Chronicles of Narnia, with its wardrobe that led to an alternate universe. Which of course is also in other hugely successful stories like Neil Gaiman's work and Eden Robinson's Trickster books. Here's the thing: Frances Hodgson Burnett, the author of *The Secret Garden*, was always writing about mental health. As a person who suffered from depression and insomnia, she turned to what was available at the time that was not "bed rest," the "cure" most often given to women suffering from what was known as "weak nerves" and encompassed everything from anxiety to migraines. Looking to Christian Science, Burnett believed in the power of positive thinking and how keeping positive self stories, like how we are a part of the natural world, can impact your overall wellness. Of course, there's so much more to being well, and what is considered mental health goes beyond just having pretty thoughts, and I can't begin to understand Christian Science, but I do know that it can't hurt to feel connected, to have good stories to bookend the more morose ones.

I loved this book for more than the idea that just beyond the next wall, just through the next gate, there might be something magical, something just for me, especially because I couldn't help but pay attention to everything in the dark. I loved it because the children in the book broke free from expectations (which in the late 1800s were apparently to be quiet and not ask questions, to stay very still). I loved it because they believed in themselves, in the positive possibility of themselves.

THE CELEBRATION OF YOU

I just finished writing a different manuscript (I had a very busy pandemic) about a thirteen-year-old girl. By the end, for her happily ever after, she decides that she will always choose herself. That she will write the most beautiful story she can think of—the story of herself. The initial feedback from the editor was that those thoughts, that section, needed to go; those lines should be cut because it made her seem like a narcissist—selfish. And I fought back.

Everything else in life tells us to put everyone before ourselves. That to become the protagonist it is ONLY by giving all we have for others that we can achieve greatness. And while this is important, for sure, especially in a community, you cannot leave yourself out of that equation. We cannot be self-effacing when we also have to be strong enough to stand up. I needed my character and every thirteen-year-old who read about her to know that it was okay to choose yourself. To consciously choose yourself. You are an important part of the community and therefore you also need the care that they need.

Lee Maracle used to always talk about this. She explained that celebrating yourself, holding your hard work and successes up, meant that your community then had the opportunity to celebrate and hold up. That being great was a gift to your family, your community, and your ancestors. Once at an event that my colleague and I had organized, she asked us to stand up so we could be acknowledged. We tried to demure, insisting the event was to celebrate her and other Elders and teachers—all their work. Lee made sure we stood up, explaining, "When you give us a chance to celebrate you, we have a chance to celebrate ourselves, the result of all that work we did, so that you COULD stand here." I remember that every time I am called to a stage.

It feels like sometimes staying small, not speaking up or celebrating your wins, is a way to be safe. Especially with social media and the way bullying has become normalized. It's easier if no one notices you and turns their negativity towards you. It also may feel like, *Well, if I do all the worrying myself, if I carefully consider what could have gone wrong and the ways this isn't that great, then that's covered.* You might feel like you did it and now no one can further tear you down. As if disaster floats above looking for bright shiny things that are untainted by doubt to swoop in. And that by tainting your own bright shininess with doubt, that disaster will float right on by. That is a horror story and it's not true—it's just living through the horribleness once for sure, because you've made sure it happens, and potentially twice.

RUPAUL'S PRESENT

Anyone who knows me knows that I love RuPaul. There is even a RuPaul quote in *Hunting by Stars*—seriously. No one has called me on it, but it's there. RuPaul often says, "It's none of my business what other people think of me." How liberating is that? Not only do you not have to care about how others define you, but that, in fact, it is not even something you should do. This is not to say we are not community people; instead, it invites us as community people to live our best lives without giving extra weight to others' impressions, which, in turn, frees them up to be responsible for their own thoughts.

But one of my favourite RuPaul quotes of all times doesn't come from *Drag Race*; it comes from his MasterClass. In it he explains that we are stars and our only job is to shine. And when we do our job, the universe is pleased. Things are right. Shining attracts more light to us. He also suggests that stressing about what has happened in the past (say, at two in the morning) and worrying about what might happen in the future (the other shoe dropping) is not living. He says, "If you've got one foot in the past, and one foot in the future, then you're just pissing on the present."

HOW WE BEGIN

The best thing I can give myself as a person who suffers with acute anxiety is unconditional love. And that seems easy to say, but it has been almost impossible to practice. Unconditional—without conditions. So that means not torturing myself by blowing up past issues and future potentials into full-colour nightmare tapestries that cover every surface. That means not ignoring the signs that I am doing too much with too few resources (time, rest, joy), which then leads to fear and loathing, trying to hold onto and be accountable for every second when I was moving too fast to be hypervigilant. The best thing I can do is to remember the anthology is full and broken and beautiful and hard and that it's all mine—it is a full banquet. And that I can take from it the nutrition that I need in any moment. Even better, sometimes the best thing you can do is to put down the anthology and just live. That's a great beginning.

Every time we celebrate ourselves, sing the song of ourselves, write the story of us, that is a story for the anthology. That is the context we need so that when we flip through our book, we have context and light. We read hilarity and a return from darkness. We see ourselves.

Thank you for letting me tell this story. This story has been one of the better stories I've told in my competition with anxiety. This story has changed the scoreboard in our favour. This story is one I will remember at two and three and four in the morning, lying in my bed, wondering what comes next.

CLC KREISEL LECTURE SERIES

Published by University of Alberta Press and the
Canadian Literature Centre / Centre de littérature canadienne